Contents

Part Two: High risk patients

Reforming The Mental Health Act

Part II:
High risk patients

Presented to Parliament by the Secretary of State for Health
and the Home Secretary by Command of Her Majesty – December 2000

Cm 5016–II

Cover Price £14.20

2 Volumes – not to be sold separately

© **Crown Copyright 2000**

Executive summary

1   This White Paper sets out the Government's proposals for improving and modernising services for people with mental health problems. This will be achieved through new legislative powers, new resources and new national standards for care and treatment in the Mental Health National Service Framework. The vast majority of these people pose no threat to others and, in many cases, are among the most vulnerable in society. But in a minority of cases, people with mental health problems may pose a serious threat to the safety of others.

2   Public protection is one of the Government's highest priorities. Public protection and the modernisation of mental health powers and services are complementary aims. New, more transparent powers, clearer pathways and processes, and more resources for specialist services will both provide greater protection to the public and improve the quality of services for the individuals themselves. Part One of this White paper sets out the Government's proposals for change to the Mental Health Act. This part of the White Paper shows how these changes will operate for the high risk group within the context of extra resources for improved specialist services.

Patients who pose a significant risk of serious harm to others

3   The vast majority of people treated under mental health legislation are treated in their own best interests, in many cases to protect them from self-harm. By contrast, there are a smaller number of people with mental disorder who are characterised by the risk that they present to others. This group includes a very small number of people detained under civil powers, and others who are remanded or convicted offenders.

4   Within this wider group are a number of individuals whose risk is as a result of a severe personality disorder. A narrow interpretation of the definition of the 'treatability' provision in the 1983 Act, together with a lack of dedicated provision within existing services, means that current arrangements for this group are inadequate both to protect the public and to provide the individuals themselves with the high quality services they need.

The criteria

5   New criteria for compulsory treatment under the Act will form a key part of these changes. These criteria will provide clear authority for the detention for assessment and treatment of all those who pose a significant risk of serious harm to others as a result of a mental disorder. The criteria will achieve this by dealing separately with those who need treatment primarily in their own best interests and those who need treatment because of the risk that they pose to others. In high risk cases, the use of compulsory

powers will be linked to the availability of a treatment plan needed either to treat the underlying mental disorder or to manage behaviours arising from the disorder.

Assessment

6   Legislation must also respond to the various ways in which such individuals come to the notice of statutory agencies. The White Paper sets out the processes for initial and more detailed assessment for such high risk individuals in the community. In some cases, these people will already be under the supervision of the probation service. Others may be known to mental health or social services or may come to the notice of the police in the course of their work. Powers in the Criminal Justice and Court Services Act 2000, expected to be implemented in April 2001, will mean that the police and probation services will be under a new statutory duty to assess and manage relevant sexual or violent offenders. Under new mental health legislation, the relevant statutory agencies will be able to refer the individual for an initial assessment and, if the initial criteria are satisfied, apply for a 28 day period of compulsory care and treatment to allow for more detailed assessment. Beyond 28 days, compulsory care must be authorised by a new independent decision making body – the Mental Health Tribunal – which will obtain advice from independent experts as well as taking evidence from the clinical team, the patient and his or her representatives, and other agencies, where appropriate.

7   These arrangements will be sufficiently flexible both to provide for the immediate healthcare needs of individuals and to ensure that they are kept in the appropriate degree of security. In addition to existing facilities, specialist assessment facilities for those who are dangerous and severely personality disordered (DSPD) are being established for the in-depth assessment needed for this group.

8   Arrangements for the assessment of those already serving prison sentences will also be improved by the creation of a new power for the Home Secretary to direct such individuals for assessment. In the case of those who may be DSPD, these assessments could be carried out in specialist facilities in either the Prison Service or the NHS.

9   For those before the Courts for an offence, there will be a new single power for the Court to remand for assessment and treatment.

Treatment

10   Under new legislation, the Tribunal – or the Court in the case of mentally disordered offenders – will be able to make a care and treatment order which will authorise the care and treatment specified in a care plan recommended by the clinical team. This must be designed to give therapeutic benefit to the patient or to manage behaviour associated with mental disorder that might lead to serious harm to other people. The first two orders will be for up to 6 months each; subsequent orders may be for periods of up to 12 months. Where treatment is authorised under the legislation, individuals will be transferred to appropriate NHS facilities taking account of any security risks that they pose. Wherever possible, treatment will be specifically aimed at addressing the underlying mental disorder. But in all high risk cases, treatment will be designed both to manage the consequences of a mental disorder as well as to enable the individuals themselves to work towards successful re-integration into the community.

Safeguards and oversight

11   The Government is committed to ensuring that any new arrangements are fully compliant with the Human Rights Act 1998. The White Paper sets out safeguards and protections for those to be detained under the Act. These will apply equally to this high risk group. The introduction of a requirement that all longer-term care and treatment orders are authorised by a body independent of the clinical team is a key way in which the new legislation will protect patient rights. But all those detained under compulsory powers will also have the right to:

- free legal representation;

- access to independent specialist advocacy services; and,

- provisions to cover the use of certain specified treatments for mental disorder and all long-term treatment without consent.

12   The White Paper also sets out new arrangements for the oversight of the new legislation and for the provision of annual reports through the creation of a new Commission for Mental Health.

Developing services for those who are DSPD

13   However, in the case of those who are dangerous as a result of a severe personality disorder, legislative changes alone are not enough. New powers must be backed up by a programme of service development that will begin to provide the capacity and specialist approaches to treatment and assessment that this group needs. Resources allocated within the recent Spending Review across the Department of Health, Home Office and Prison Service include an additional £126m over the next three years for the development of new specialist services for those who are high risk as a result of a severe personality disorder.

14   The Government recognises the importance of building a secure evidence-base for these services and is therefore committed to a series of pilot projects to test out new approaches. The assessment process is already being piloted in both NHS and Prison Service high security settings and the first treatment pilots will begin in 2001. These pilot projects will be rigorously and independently evaluated as part of a comprehensive research agenda.

15   Capacity for the pilots will be created through a programme of refurbishing existing accommodation and new builds. Over the next three years this will provide:

- 320 additional specialist places across the Prison Service and the NHS; and,

- 75 hostel places.

The pilots will also inform subsequent decisions on the nature, scale and pace of any further expansion of services beyond this first phase.

Sharing information

16   Improved public protection also relies on the effective co-operation of the various statutory agencies. The Criminal Justice and Court Services Act 2000 has already placed a new statutory duty on police and probation services to establish arrangements for

assessing and managing the risks posed by relevant sexual and violent dangerous offenders. In respect of those who are mentally disordered, new mental health legislation will build on this approach by introducing a new duty covering the disclosure of information about patients suffering from mental disorder between health and social services agencies and other agencies, for example housing agencies or criminal justice agencies.

17 We will also introduce new arrangements for the provision of information to victims of mentally disordered offenders who have committed serious violent or sexual offences and who have been given a care and treatment order by the Courts rather than a prison sentence.

Chapter One

Mental disorder and public protection

Introduction

1.1 This second part of the White Paper sets out new arrangements for managing people who need to be detained and treated under Mental Health Act powers because of the high level of risk that they pose to others as a result of their mental disorder. The arrangements form part of wider changes to the powers for compulsory care and treatment and the delivery of mental health services that are set out in the first part of this White Paper. For a comprehensive picture, both parts of the White Paper will need to be read.

1.2 Alongside changes to legal provisions, this part of the White Paper also sets out the changes already underway to improve specialist secure mental health services, which will be required to ensure the delivery of high quality services to patients and to facilitate the proper implementation of the new powers. The Government believes that where individuals are deprived of their liberty because of their mental disorder, they should be provided with high quality mental health services delivered in an appropriate environment.

Who are we talking about?

1.3 The vast majority of people who currently receive treatment for a mental disorder under the Mental Health Act 1983 do not pose a risk to others. They are detained in their own best interests, in many cases to protect them from self-harm. By contrast, there is a smaller number of individuals with mental disorder with whom this paper is concerned who are characterised primarily by the risk that they present to others. This latter group will include both those detained under civil powers, and those mentally disordered offenders who have been given a mental health disposal and a restriction order under Part III of the Mental Health Act 1983.

1.4 These patients detained under the Mental Health Act 1983 are currently managed in a range of specialist secure mental health services, including high security services. The 1983 Act does not however provide any particular statutory provisions to govern the care and treatment of this high risk group apart from the restriction order for mentally disordered offenders. Under new mental health legislation, there will be a single set of criteria and processes which will apply to all mental disorders but within this overarching framework, there will be specific recognition of the fact that for some people their plan of care and treatment will be primarily designed to manage and reduce high risk behaviours which pose a significant risk to others. The new legislation will balance the rights of the patient who is undergoing compulsory care and treatment with the right of the public to be protected from serious harm.

Dangerous People with Severe Personality Disorder

1.5 Among this group there are a number of individuals who pose a significant risk of serious harm to others as a result of their severe personality disorder. The consultation paper *Managing Dangerous People with Severe Personality Disorder*[1] set out our proposals to deal more effectively with the risk this group poses. As set out in the consultation paper, work carried out by the Office for National Statistics on the prison population[2], together with an analysis of those detained in secure hospitals, and community estimates, suggests that a total of between 2,100 and 2,400 men are dangerous and severely personality disordered (DSPD). Further work is now underway to refine these estimates and to include women who are DSPD.

1.6 Chapter Two summarises the responses to the consultation paper and describes the way forward now proposed. Chapters Three and Four include a description of how the provisions of the new mental health legislation will apply to the DSPD group. The legal provisions that apply will be the same for all those who are assessed as posing a risk to others as a result of their mental disorder, whatever the diagnosis, but they will contain some flexibility which allows for the different processes of assessment that are proposed for those who are thought to be DSPD. Chapter Six includes the programme of DSPD service development that is already underway.

How these proposals link to the Government's objectives and priorities

1.7 These proposals form an important part of the delivery of two of the Government's key priorities:

- **public protection** – the public rightly demand protection from the risks posed by dangerous people in society;

- **modernising the NHS** – the provision of high quality, efficient services which are evidence-based and responsive to need.

Public protection

1.8 There is no single answer to the problem of dangerousness. No society can ever be completely free of the risk of serious harm. But where there are deficiencies in the law and in the provision of specialist services – as in the case of those who are dangerous and severely personality disordered – the public rightly expects the Government to take action. These proposals do not provide the only response to the various weaknesses in the law that the Government has identified. They are a specific solution to a particular problem which address the risks posed by those whose behaviour stems from their mental disorder. But they are an important part of a wider package of changes which includes:

- legislative measures requiring sex offenders to register with the police on leaving prison under the Sex Offenders Act 1997, Sex Offender Orders introduced under the Crime and Disorder Act 1998 and the automatic life sentence for a second serious violent or sexual offence under the Crime (Sentences) Act 1997;

- an 'Early Warning System' to alert the Home Office to the imminent release of potentially dangerous violent or sexual offenders and enable the risk management arrangements for those offenders to be monitored.

[1] Managing Dangerous People with Severe Personality Disorder. Proposals for Policy Development. Home Office/Department of Health. July 1999.

[2] Psychiatric Morbidity among prisoners in England and Wales. Office for National Statistics. 1998.

The Government is also developing further measures to:

- strengthen the effectiveness and protection of the law for children;

- put police and probation service risk management arrangements on a statutory basis to improve standards;

- prevent offenders who have committed offences of sex or violence against children from working with them on release;

- electronically monitor dangerous offenders as a licence condition.

Modernising mental health services

1.9 In the same way, these proposals are a part of a much broader Government strategy to improve the quality and consistency of health and social services for people who suffer from mental health problems, as set out in *Modernising Mental Health Services*[3] (and which is being taken forward in Wales in the emerging All Wales strategy[4]) and *The NHS Plan*[5]. In addition, the *National Service Framework for Mental Health*[6] has established for the first time, new national standards of care and treatment of mental disorder. This has been backed by significant additional funding to provide better and faster care for those who need treatment and support.

1.10 Modern mental health legislation is required to support these service changes, to protect the rights of patients and the public, to enhance the principles of fairness and equity and ensure consistency in the application of compulsory powers.

Safeguards to protect patients

1.11 New legislation will be fully compliant with the Human Rights Act 1998. The processes for the application of compulsory powers in the new legislation are designed to enhance the rights of patients. In particular, the introduction of a requirement that all longer-term care and treatment orders are authorised by a body independent of the clinical team is a key way in which the new legislation will protect patient rights.

1.12 In addition, Chapter Five of Part One of this White Paper sets out a number of specific provisions that will be contained within new legislation to safeguard the rights of patients who are subject to compulsory care and treatment. These include:

- access to independent specialist advocacy services;

- provisions to cover the use of certain specified treatments for mental disorder and all long-term treatment without consent.

1.13 All these safeguards will apply equally to all those who are subject to compulsory powers, regardless of whether they are subject to compulsory powers on the basis of the risk of significant harm that they pose to others or because it is in their own best interests. As now, all patients will also have a right to free legal representation.

[3] Modernising Mental Health Services: Safe, sound and supportive. Department of Health. December 1998.

[4] TSO 1998 Cm 4169.

[5] The NHS Plan: A plan for investment, a plan for reform. Department of Health. July 2000.

[6] Mental Health National Service Framework. Department of Health. September 1999.

Oversight of the new legislation

1.14 The new legislation will make provision for the Secretary of State to establish a Commission for Mental Health. The Commission will take on many of the functions of the current Mental Health Act Commission (see Part One, paragraph 7.8), but with a fresh emphasis on monitoring the implementation of the safeguards which ensure that compulsory powers are properly used. Issues of the quality and consistency of services provided, such as the nature of the environment, access to fresh air and activities, and visiting arrangements will fall within the remit of the Commission for Health Improvement or the National Care Standards Commission.

1.15 The Commission will consist of a primarily non-executive Board with a non-executive Chairman and members representative of users, carers and the key professional bodies. Key executive staff of the Commission will also be members of the Board. The Commission will be required to provide the Secretary of State with an annual report on its work that will be made public. (See Part One, paragraph 7.6)

Chapter Two

Managing Dangerous People with Severe Personality Disorder

Introduction

2.1 The consultation paper *Managing Dangerous People with Severe Personality Disorder*[7], published in July 1999, set out the Government's proposals for tackling the challenge to public safety presented by the very small minority of people with severe personality disorder, who because of their disorder, pose a high risk of serious offending. There are two key elements to these proposals:

- to ensure that dangerous people with severe personality disorder are kept in detention for as long as they pose a high risk to others; and,

- to provide high quality services to enable them to deal with the consequences of their disorder, reduce their risk to others and so work towards successful re-integration into the community.

The problem

2.2 Successive Governments have grappled with the problems posed by people who are DSPD. At present neither mental health nor criminal justice legislation deals adequately with the risks this group pose to the public. In many cases, an individual who is DSPD has to be released from prison at the end of a determinate sentence even though they are assessed as presenting a continuing risk of harm to others. Individuals who present a risk to others because of their severe personality disorder are rarely detained under the Mental Health Act 1983 because they are assessed as being unlikely to benefit from the sorts of treatment currently available in hospital.

2.3 The deficiencies in the law are accompanied by a lack of specialist provision for the assessment and treatment of this group. Until now, a lack of strategic direction has meant little progress in developing a robust long term solution to this problem.

The Government's proposals

2.4 The consultation paper described two possible approaches. **Option A** built on existing service structures and makes changes to existing powers of detention – both criminal justice and mental health powers. **Option B** proposed the creation of a new service and new civil and criminal powers for the detention of this group, including powers for supervision and recall following detention.

[7] Managing Dangerous People with Severe Personality Disorder. Proposals for Policy Development. Home Office/Department of Health. July 1999.

Option A

- amends criminal justice legislation to allow for greater use of **discretionary life sentences**;

- amends Mental Health Act 1983 **to remove the 'treatability criterion'** for civil detainees;

- services continue to be provided in specialist facilities in both prisons and secure mental health services.

Option B

- new powers in civil and criminal proceedings for indeterminate detention of DSPD individuals (including powers for supervision and recall following detention);

- individuals held in a new service separately managed from mainstream prison and health services – the 'third service'.

The consultation process

2.5 The consultation paper marked the beginning of a major debate about the most effective and ethical ways of dealing with this group. We received 290 responses. Many of these were from organisations representing a large number of constituents who had themselves carried out extensive internal consultation. A broad range of views was put forward. Whilst those who responded overwhelmingly agreed that present arrangements were inadequate, there was disagreement as to how best to proceed.

2.6 Of those expressing a preference between the two options, the majority preferred Option B in the long term, though there was some concern about aspects of these proposals. The main opposition, on civil liberty grounds, was to the proposal to detain in civil cases. In part, concerns were based on what we believe are misplaced fears about the nature of the proposals and their scope. It was wrongly suggested that these proposals were about the widespread detention of all those who may have suffered from a personality disorder – however mild – or whose offending history meant that they may have posed a risk to others at some point in the past. Concerns were also expressed about:

- the absence of dedicated specialist services and fears that any individual detained under new powers would be held in unsuitable conditions;

- our ability – with our current knowledge – accurately to assess and diagnose such individuals and subsequently to manage them safely in a suitable therapeutic environment which enables them to work towards a successful re-integration into the community.

2.7 However, despite these concerns, it was generally felt that the high quality services required for this group were more likely to be achieved under Option B.

2.8 Respondents welcomed the Government's emphasis on research and in particular the need for further research into risk assessment processes and treatment. There was general support for a multi-disciplinary approach to the assessment and treatment of this group and recognition that specialist training for a multi-disciplinary workforce is essential.

2.9 During the consultation period, we also enlisted the help of 70 experts and practitioners in the mental health and criminal justice systems to examine the practical details of the assessment process that will underpin new arrangements. A key aspect of this work has been the development of an assessment process, which is being piloted in high security settings in both the NHS and the Prison Service. The proposals will also feed into the pilot projects and the research agenda as new services are developed, for example, proposals to ensure that assessment processes are non-discriminatory and take full account of the special needs of those from ethnic minority communities, women, and those suffering from co-existing mental illness or problems relating to drug or alcohol misuse.

2.10 We have taken account of the House of Commons Home Affairs Committee Report published on 14 March 2000, which unanimously supported the proposals, and the views of the Health Select Committee, who published their Report into NHS Mental Health Services on 24 July 2000, as well as the large number of debates and conferences prompted by the proposals.

Cost benefit analysis

2.11 A cost benefit analysis was carried out to model the treatment and detention of those who are dangerous and severely personality disordered under the two options set out in the consultation paper. This analysis provided a very broad indication of the likely scale of costs under both options because of uncertainties about, for example, the numbers of those who will be assessed as being dangerous and severely personality disordered, the effectiveness of treatment and therefore the average length of detention, and the precise number of staff and mix of skills required. In order to refine these costs, further work is therefore required over the piloting period to clarify these issues. This work will form an important part of the research strategy and will be made public when it is available.

The way forward

2.12 The Government has decided that before taking final decisions on how best to provide services for this group in the long term, it needs to pilot and evaluate the assessment process and the various treatments available for this group within existing service structures. At the same time, we will bring forward those legislative changes that will be required whether Option A or Option B is adopted. Our proposals for reform of the Mental Health Act 1983 will provide a new framework of powers which will provide for the detention of dangerous people with severe personality disorder in a therapeutic environment for as long as they pose a risk to others as a result of their mental disorder.

2.13 Because these powers will be based on the presence of a mental disorder new powers for detention will apply to individuals in civil proceedings, as well as to those being sentenced for an offence. But in practice, the nature of the assessment process means that it is highly unlikely that any individual without a long track record of increasingly serious offending will be affected by these new powers. The Government is committed to ensuring that any new powers are fully compatible with the Human Rights Act 1998, and proper safeguards have been developed as part of these proposals.

2.14 Chapters Three and Four of this part of the White Paper describe the new powers in mental health legislation and how they will be applied to the DSPD group. Chapter Six includes a description of how specialist DSPD services will be organised and developed in both the NHS and the prison service over the next three years, in order to ensure that by the end of the period the Government is well placed to take longer term decisions.

2.15 Our proposals set out in this White Paper, and the sequencing of their introduction provide a practical way of making progress on these issues of concern whilst also addressing the fundamental challenge of public protection. This is not a problem which can be solved in its entirety at a stroke. It will require years of research, service development, specialist staff training, work to determine the best possible environmental setting and most effective treatments before we can be sure that we have the most effective services for this group. Indeed we can always improve services and knowledge. But that cannot be a reason to fail now to embark on the process or to take powers which are needed to protect the public.

Managing the programme of change

2.16 These changes cannot be accomplished without the co-operation of a wide group of stakeholders in this process. We have established an inter-departmental programme which brings together officials from the Department of Health, the Prison Service and the Home Office working as part of a single team to co-ordinate every aspect of these changes. Distinct projects have been established to cover:

- treatment and assessment;

- human resources and training;

- construction;

- legislation;

- women's services;

- community services;

- research and development.

These are underpinned by a communication project and a project to enable proper business planning for the expansion of services.

2.17 These projects also involve a great many external stakeholders but especially managers, clinicians and practitioners in the NHS and the Prison Service, academics and the research community. Many of these are involved in the various project teams and supporting advisory groups. We are committed to working in partnership with these and other groups to ensure that services and powers are developed which can be used effectively on the ground.

Definitions

2.18 It should be stressed that the phrase 'dangerous people with severe personality disorder' is a working definition. It is designed to cover individuals who:

- show significant disorder of personality;

- present a significant risk of causing serious physical or psychological harm from which the victim would find it difficult or impossible to recover, e.g. homicide, rape, arson; and in whom,

- the risk presented appears to be functionally linked to the personality disorder.

We intend to refine this definition during the pilot period as we develop a clearer picture of the nature and characteristics of this group.

Chapter Three

New statutory powers for the assessment and treatment of high risk patients in civil proceedings

Criteria for compulsory care and treatment

3.1 Chapter Three of Part One of this White Paper sets out the criteria which will clearly define the limits of compulsory powers.

3.2 Powers in the new legislation will be based on a broad definition of mental disorder covering any disability or disorder of mind or brain, whether permanent or temporary, which results in an impairment or disturbance of mental functioning. No categories of mental disorder will be defined in the legislation. This approach will ensure the flexibility for formal powers to be used in whatever way best meets a particular patient's needs and is consistent with any risk that they pose to themselves or to other people. One of the effects of the change will be to move away from the narrow concept of 'treatability' that applies to certain categories of mental disorder in the 1983 Act.

3.3 A preliminary examination will, generally, be carried out by two doctors and a social worker, or another mental health professional with specific training in the application of the new legislation, to confirm whether it is appropriate to use compulsory powers. The assessment will be on the basis that there are reasonable grounds to believe that the patient is suffering from a mental disorder that is sufficiently serious to warrant further assessment or urgent treatment by specialist mental health services, and that, without such intervention, the patient is likely to be at risk of serious harm, including deterioration in health, or pose a significant risk of serious harm to other people.

3.4 Once the decision to use compulsory powers has been confirmed, the care team will be required to prepare a preliminary written care plan within 3 days. Care and treatment under formal powers will only be able to be continued after the first 3 days if clear criteria are met. The criteria will cover three related issues:

- the patient must be diagnosed as suffering from a mental disorder within the meaning of the new legislation;

- the mental disorder must be of a nature or degree as to warrant specialist care and treatment. This may be necessary in the best interests of the patient and/or because without care and treatment there is a significant risk of serious harm to other people;

- a plan of care and treatment must be available to address the mental disorder. In cases where the use of compulsory powers arises primarily in the patient's own best interests, that plan must be anticipated to be of direct therapeutic benefit to the individual concerned. In cases where compulsory powers are sought primarily because of the risk that the patient poses to others, the plan must be considered necessary either directly to treat the underlying mental disorder and/or to manage behaviours arising from the disorder.

3.5 The initial period of assessment and treatment under compulsory powers will be limited to a maximum of 28 days. After that period, continuing use of compulsory powers must be authorised by a new independent decision making body – the new Mental Health Tribunal. There will be provision for a fast track procedure to allow a case to be referred to the Tribunal for review before 28 days.

Managing high risk individuals with mental disorder

3.6 Compulsory care and treatment may be necessary to manage behaviours arising from the mental disorder that may lead to serious harm to other people. In such cases, where a person is subject to compulsory care and treatment on the basis of the risk they pose to others, the care plan must include the provision of interventions that are specifically designed to ameliorate the behaviours that cause them to be a risk to others.

3.7 This approach will provide greater transparency for both patients and those applying the new legislation. The new provisions are designed to allow for a flexible approach to the management of high risk individuals depending on the type of specialist service they require, the degree to which their underlying mental disorder can be 'treated' and where specialist care and treatment can best be provided.

Managing Dangerous People with Severe Personality Disorder – The Criteria

The new criteria for the application of provisions for compulsory care and treatment are designed to provide a comprehensive description of those patients who should come within the remit of mental health legislation, and remove some of the current difficulties present in the criteria in the 1983 Act. The requirement of 'treatability' in the 1983 Act for those falling in the category of psychopathic disorder or mental impairment is unhelpful and has neither met the needs of patients nor helped to give the public the protection it needs. The new legislation will address this problem.

Powers under new legislation will be able to be applied to an individual who poses a significant risk of serious harm to others as a result of their mental disorder including where a plan of care and treatment appropriate to that person is considered necessary to manage behaviours arising from mental disorder that may lead to serious harm to other people (see paragraph 3.4 above). In all cases, care and treatment must be delivered in an appropriate therapeutic environment.

This approach will provide the unambiguous authority to detain individuals who would fall within the DSPD group where appropriate interventions are offered to tackle the individual's high risk behaviour.

Assessment for use of compulsory powers

3.8 A preliminary examination will be required before a patient is made subject to compulsory powers (see paragraph 3.3 above). It will be a requirement of the initial application for use of compulsory powers for an initial period of 28 days that all assessments under the new legislation should include consideration of the risk that the patient poses to others.

3.9 Once the patient is made subject to compulsory powers, there will follow a period of further formal assessment (although if the patient is already known to the service this may be very short). During this time, a more in-depth assessment of the risk that the patient might pose to others will take place, including consideration of evidence from criminal justice agencies, if appropriate. This in-depth assessment is necessary before a suitable care plan can be drawn up. Consideration of the risk the patient poses would also influence decisions on the level of security the patient requires during in-patient treatment.

Referral by criminal justice agencies in the community for an assessment

3.10 Increasingly, criminal justice agencies are working together to manage the risk posed by potentially dangerous offenders in the community. Until now, these arrangements have been informal, flowing from the requirements of the Sex Offenders Act 1997. In many cases, health, social services and housing agencies have been invited to join local 'multi-agency risk panels' or 'public protection panels' to provide expertise and support to the police and probation services in the supervision and monitoring of high risk individuals with mental disorder (whether or not a formal mental health assessment has been carried out).

3.11 The Government has recently put local risk management arrangements on a statutory footing by requiring police and probation services to draw up local risk management strategies. These provisions have been included within the Criminal Justice and Court Services Act 2000 (see paragraphs 5.4 – 5.6) and are expected to come into force in April 2001.

3.12 It will be important for processes in new mental health legislation to provide for a swift response to concerns about supervised and monitored high risk individuals from all members of the multi-agency risk panel, particularly those with a statutory duty to manage high risk individuals in the community. There will therefore be a statutory duty on the relevant NHS trust or Primary Care Trust that is responsible for providing specialist mental health services in the area to undertake a preliminary examination when receiving applications from the police and the probation services. (This duty will also extend to the patient's GP, the Courts, the Prison Service and the patient's carer – see Chapter Three of Part One).

Managing Dangerous People with Severe Personality Disorder – Case Study 'A'

A is currently living in bed and breakfast accommodation and is supervised by the probation service. She has a history of setting fires and convictions for theft and arson; during previous periods in detention she has assaulted staff. She has no family contact. Her most recent offence resulted in the death of her victim. She was held on remand and then assessed for treatment of her personality disorder under the Mental Health Act 1983, but considered 'untreatable' given currently available services. The Courts imposed a determinate prison sentence and she is now on licence in the community having served the custodial part of the sentence without parole. She is a compulsive self harmer and emotionally unstable. She presents a risk to herself and others, having made suicide attempts in the past and is unwilling to engage in meaningful dialogue with the agencies to get to the roots of her present situation and behaviour.

The probation service would be able to refer A for assessment under the new mental health legislation. A DSPD screening assessment could be carried out in the community, but A's unsettled lifestyle may indicate that she should be detained in a suitable NHS facility for an initial examination. If further intensive assessment was indicated, she would be transferred to a specialist NHS DSPD assessment facility and at 28 days the Mental Health Tribunal would be asked to authorise a further period of specialist assessment. A care and treatment plan would then be drawn up which would be delivered in an appropriate therapeutic environment within the NHS.

Police powers to remove to a place of safety and seek assessment in an emergency

3.13 There will continue to be a power for the police to remove a person from a public place if he or she appears to be suffering from a mental disorder and in need of care and control. In some cases, individuals may be required to be removed by the police where they are posing an immediate risk of harm to the public because of violent or threatening behaviour (see paragraphs 3.79-3.85 in Part One).

The Mental Health Tribunal and high risk patients

3.14 Chapter Three of Part One of the Paper describes the composition and operation of the new Mental Health Tribunal in civil proceedings.

3.15 The new Mental Health Tribunal is designed to provide independent scrutiny of all proposals to continue care and treatment under compulsory powers for longer than 28 days. Continuing care and treatment will be based on recommendations from the patient's clinical supervisor but will need to be authorised by the Tribunal.

3.16 The Tribunal will have a legally qualified chair and two other members with experience of mental health services. One of the members will be a person with a clinical background and the other will usually have a background in community or voluntary sector service provision. Before continuing care and treatment beyond the initial 28 day period is authorised, the patient will be seen by an independent doctor drawn from a panel of people appointed to provide expert evidence to the Tribunal. Wherever possible the medical expert who sees the patient will have expertise in the particular type of mental disorder from which he or she is suffering.

3.17 Where a compulsory care and treatment order is sought by the clinical supervisor on the basis of the significant risk of serious harm that the patient poses to others, the medical expert will generally have a background in forensic psychiatry or psychology.

3.18 On the first two occasions that the Tribunal hears an application from the clinical supervisor, it will be able to make a care and treatment order that lasts for up to 6 months. Subsequent orders may be for up to 12 months at a time. The patient will be able to request a review of their care and treatment once during the period of an order which lasts longer than 3 months. This review will not constitute an appeal against the original order but will determine whether the current arrangements for compulsory care and treatment are appropriate.

3.19 The Tribunal will have a power to call before it anyone else whom it sees as relevant. Criminal justice and other agencies involved in formal risk management arrangements in the community (see paragraph 3.10 − 3.11 above) will be able to provide evidence of risk to others from the individual before the Tribunal, which would be independent of the assessment by the clinical team. This may include evidence of previous criminal behaviour, and would be particularly useful where this shows a pattern of increasingly serious offending. The Tribunal will have a duty to consider all such evidence in making its decision.

Tribunal authority to discharge, grant leave or vary the conditions of the care and treatment order in civil proceedings for high risk patients

3.20 In most cases, decisions to discharge a patient from detention in hospital or to vary certain conditions of the order, for example, by transferring the patient to another hospital, will be taken by the clinical supervisor.

3.21 Exceptionally, the Tribunal will be able to require that decisions on discharge, leave and transfer should be referred to it for prior approval. This would usually be appropriate where someone has been subject to a compulsory care and treatment order in a secure hospital on the basis of the risk of harm they pose to others as a result of their mental disorder. This provision will allow the Tribunal to continue independently to scrutinise the evidence of risk to others from both the clinical team, and other agencies, before the patient is discharged from detention in hospital, or significant changes are made to the care plan. Changes to the care plan might include transfer to conditions of lesser security, or the granting of leave at home.

Discharge of high risk patients

3.22 Patients detained in hospital on the basis of the risk they pose to others will only be discharged into the community following a comprehensive risk assessment which demonstrates that risk has been reduced. It is anticipated that for the majority of such patients, a period of rehabilitation in the community will be required under the supervision of community mental health services. In most of these cases, it is expected that discharge from detention in hospital will be followed by a period of compulsory care and treatment in the community. A care and treatment order in the community would include specific requirements and would specify what action the clinical supervisor is empowered to take if the patient fails to comply, including a provision for recall to hospital. Recall to hospital would also be effected where the care and treatment the patient required could no longer be given effectively or safely in the community, or where the patient's continued presence in the community would pose a risk of serious harm to others.

3.23 Supervision whilst on a community treatment order may include the involvement of the local multi-agency risk management panel, where their involvement is thought appropriate in the circumstances of the case.

Managing Dangerous People with Severe Personality Disorder – Assessment in Civil Proceedings

A small number of individuals in the community may pose a significant risk of serious harm to others as a result of their severe personality disorder. The majority will have been previously convicted of a serious violent or sexual offence and some will be under the supervision of the probation service. If they are thought to present a continuing risk to the public they will be subject to local risk management arrangements led by the police and probation services (see paragraphs 3.10 and 3.11 and paragraphs 5.4 – 5.6). In some cases such individuals will come to the notice of local mental health services or social services.

Where criminal justice agencies have concerns about the risk an individual poses to others as a result of their personality disorder, they will be able to refer the individual for a preliminary examination under the new legislation (see paragraph 3.12 above). If the initial criteria are satisfied an application for detention in hospital for a period of 28 days will be made, and the individual will be detained initially in a suitable regional NHS secure facility for a DSPD screening assessment. In exceptional cases, the patient may be transferred immediately to a high security specialist DSPD assessment centre in the NHS if security considerations warrant it. The screening assessment will be carried out by a small specialist team including a psychiatrist and psychologist. This assessment is designed to establish whether there is sufficient evidence of someone being 'DSPD' to justify a longer term intensive assessment in a specialist assessment centre (see paragraphs 6.38 – 6.44).

In cases where a comprehensive DSPD assessment is indicated, the individual will be transferred to a specialist DSPD assessment centre within the NHS for a period of specialist assessment. The intensive assessment process is, at the moment, designed to take up to 3 months to complete (see paragraph 6.42). Once the initial period of 28 days for formal assessment has expired, or earlier if the patient applies for an expedited Tribunal, the new Mental Health Tribunal will be asked by the specialist care team carrying out the assessment to authorise a further period of detention to allow for the continuation of the intensive assessment process.

Once the assessment has been completed, a multi-disciplinary report on the patient and a comprehensive care plan, will be presented to the Mental Health Tribunal who will authorise further detention for specialist care and treatment in a specialist DSPD facility if appropriate.

Managing Dangerous People with Severe Personality Disorder – Treatment and Rehabilitation

On completion of the specialist DSPD assessment, and where the patient meets the criteria for continued detention under the new legislation, the care team will formulate a care plan for an initial phase of care and treatment which would take place in a specialist DSPD treatment facility in the NHS.

The care plan would be put before the Mental Health Tribunal to authorise a further period of detention in hospital. Because the patient will be detained primarily on the basis of the risk of harm they pose to others, the Tribunal will be able to stipulate particular conditions on the compulsory order which will allow, for example, the Tribunal to reserve the power to discharge the patient from detention in hospital.

When the patient is assessed as being ready for discharge into the community because the risk they pose to others has been significantly reduced, it is anticipated that the patient will continue to be subject to compulsory care and treatment in the community. In many cases, the patient will be discharged into a community rehabilitation hostel or similar supported accommodation. This will ensure that the patient receives appropriate ongoing care and treatment in the community, and will allow for swift recall of the patient to hospital if any of the conditions imposed are breached, or if the patient's assessed level of risk increases.

Chapter Four

Statutory powers for the assessment and treatment of high risk mentally disordered offenders

4.1 The majority of individuals who require compulsory care and treatment under powers in mental health legislation on the basis of the risk of serious harm they pose to others will be offenders, whose care and treatment is authorised by the Courts. Under new legislation, the conditions that need to be met for use of compulsory powers will be the same for mentally disordered offenders as for other people, but different procedures will apply.

4.2 Where there is a link between the offending behaviour and the person's mental disorder, compulsory care and treatment may be necessary to manage behaviours arising from the mental disorder that may lead to serious harm to other people. In the majority of cases, the care and treatment plan will also contain elements that are designed to be of direct therapeutic benefit to the individual concerned, but this will not be a requirement for a compulsory order to be imposed. (See Part One, paragraphs 3.14-3.18).

Offenders before the Courts

A single power of remand for assessment and treatment

4.3 Chapter Four of the first part of the White Paper sets out a simplified procedure for the Courts to obtain a medical assessment and order treatment at any stage of the trial when mental disorder becomes an issue.

4.4 A court remand for assessment will be based on a single medical recommendation from an appropriately qualified doctor. A second medical opinion will be required before compulsory treatment can be given. The remand could be to detention in hospital or for assessment in the community on bail. The power will apply in both magistrates' and the Higher Courts.

4.5 The order will be renewable by the Court at 28-day intervals for up to a maximum period of 12 months, on the recommendation of the clinical supervisor. But the Court will be expected to make a disposal if the person is convicted, as soon as there is sufficient information to make an effective sentencing disposal. The offender will have the right to legal representation at any hearing where renewal of the remand order or sentencing is considered.

Moving between assessment facilities

4.6 During the assessment of an offender on remand, it may be necessary to transfer the offender to a different location for specialist assessment for, for example, learning disability, or DSPD. Such changes will be ordered and reviewed by the Court on the basis of revised care and treatment plans submitted by the clinical supervisor. The offender would have the right to legal representation to contest such changes.

Agreeing leave

4.7 The remanding Court will have a power to agree to the offender being given leave from hospital on the recommendation of the clinical supervisor. In some cases, the Court will be able to allow the clinical supervisor to grant leave, but where public safety is an issue because of the nature of the offence or mental disorder, the Court itself will reserve the power to grant or refuse applications for leave.

Sentencing

4.8 Chapter Four of Part One of the White Paper sets out the range of sentencing options that will be available to the Court following a specialist assessment for mental disorder:

- **a criminal justice disposal** – this will be at the discretion of the Court to decide in the light of the offence, the medical evidence, any history of offending and the implications of a particular disposal for the offender's future management, both in terms of his or her treatment needs and any risk to other people:

  - a life sentence will be mandatory in the case of a conviction for murder; automatic in the circumstances of section 2 of the Crime Sentences Act 1997; or discretionary in the event that the offence and the evidence of the offender's dangerousness justifies it;

  - an appropriate determinate prison sentence or other criminal justice disposal could be passed.

  Any of these disposals would signal the end of detention under mental health legislation unless the Court makes a hospital direction (see below) or the person is transferred to hospital on the direction of the Home Secretary (see paragraphs 4.11 – 4.13 below).

- **a care and treatment order** – this option will be available only if, on the basis of a full assessment by specialist mental health services, the clinical supervisor recommends continuing care and treatment and the Court considers the criteria for making a care and treatment order under the new legislation are met. Unless a restriction order applies (see below) the procedures for discharge of the order would be the same as for an order made by a Mental Health Tribunal. A care and treatment order made by the Court would be for a maximum of 6 months. Any extension of liability to compulsory treatment after that would be through the procedures for a Tribunal order described in Chapter Three.

- **a restriction order** – where the clinical assessment indicates that the offender poses a significant risk of serious harm to others, or because of the nature of the current offence or previous convictions, the Court will be able to add a restriction order to a care and treatment order. This will only be applicable when the care and treatment order is based on detention in hospital.

- **a hospital and limitation direction** – the Court will retain the option of combining a criminal justice tariff with an order for care and treatment under mental health legislation by adding a hospital and limitation direction to a prison sentence. A hospital and limitation direction has the effect of requiring the offender's detention for medical treatment in hospital until such time as the clinical supervisor advises that treatment in hospital is no longer necessary. The offender can then be transferred to prison, by direction of the Home Secretary, to complete his or her sentence.

Offenders on a restriction order

4.9 The purpose of a restriction order is to ensure that decisions to grant leave, transfer or discharge the patient, or otherwise vary the order in a way that would provide greater liberty for a patient who is assessed as dangerous, are taken on the basis of a comprehensive risk assessment. Patients who are subject to restrictions will be managed under the supervision of the Home Secretary, as in the 1983 Act, and will only be able to be discharged from detention in hospital by the Mental Health Tribunal or the Home Secretary.

Hospital and limitation direction

4.10 Under new legislation this option will be available for a patient diagnosed with any mental disorder within the meaning of the legislation. The hospital direction is particularly suited to cases where care and treatment for mental disorder under compulsory powers in mental health legislation is recommended following a remand for assessment, but the nature of the offending and assessment of dangerousness indicate a need to pass a life sentence.

Managing Dangerous People with Severe Personality Disorder – Assessment and Sentencing of Offenders Before the Courts

Where an individual who may be DSPD is before the courts for an offence, it is important that judges have all the information they need to inform their sentencing decisions. Following a screening assessment, it will therefore be for the judge to order transfer of a defendant to a specialist NHS DSPD assessment centre for the full assessment process. The report of that process would then be available to the judge to assist in determining which of the various options (see paragraph 4.8 above) is appropriate. This option may come to the judge's attention in a number of ways.

Where an individual on remand for an offence is thought to have a severe personality disorder, a 'DSPD' screening assessment will be carried out by a specialist clinical team (see paragraphs 6.39 – 6.41) at the request of the prison, and the information fed back to the Court. Alternatively it may be clear to the trial judge at the beginning of the trial that a screening assessment is required. As an additional safeguard, where no screening assessment has been carried out in spite of the evidence of the high risk posed by the defendant, it will be for the responsible probation officer to consider whether to recommend a DSPD screening assessment as part of the pre-sentence report.

There will be a statutory duty on the relevant NHS trust to carry out an initial assessment under the new legislation where this has been requested by the probation service, the police, the Prison Service or the Court. If the screening assessment indicates that a specialist DSPD assessment is appropriate, the Court can direct the offender to a specialist DSPD assessment facility in the NHS for 28 days at a time whilst they remain on remand. The Court will be asked by the clinical team to renew the assessment order every 28 days until the specialist DSPD assessment is completed. The specialist DSPD assessment is currently designed to last for 3 months.

On conviction, the report from the clinical team carrying out the specialist DSPD assessment will be presented to the sentencing judge to decide on the most appropriate disposal for the offender. Where care and treatment in the NHS is indicated, a compulsory care and treatment order in hospital or hospital direction, with a limitation direction, would be recommended in the report. Where care and treatment in the NHS is not indicated, but the offender nevertheless is assessed as posing a risk of serious harm to others, the judge may consider that a discretionary life sentence, where the nature of the offence makes this an option, would be appropriate to protect the public.

Prisoners

Referral for assessment and treatment under compulsory powers

4.11 Under the 1983 Act, the Home Secretary has the power to transfer a prisoner to hospital for treatment, but does not have a power that would allow for a period of specialist assessment without treatment. The new legislation will provide for the Home Secretary to direct a prisoner to undergo a specialist assessment for mental disorder, in addition to powers to direct transfer to hospital for treatment. Such a specialist assessment will take place in an appropriate environment, which could be in a hospital, or a dedicated section of a prison. In particular, this will allow for specialist assessment of prisoners who are high risk before decisions on possible transfer to a specialist mental health unit are considered.

4.12 A transfer direction will generally specify that a prisoner is detained in hospital for treatment, and carry a restriction direction, which has the effect of a restriction order as described in paragraph 4.8 above.

4.13 When a transferred prisoner reaches the date on which he or she would have been released from prison, authorisation for continuing care and treatment will be subject to the clinical supervisor submitting an application for approval by the Mental Health Tribunal in civil proceedings as described in Chapter Three.

4.14 Where the patient remains subject to compulsory powers on expiry of their restriction direction because of the risk of harm they pose to others, the Tribunal ordering continuing care and treatment will be able to require that decisions on discharge, leave and transfer should be referred to it for prior approval. This provision will allow the Tribunal to continue independently to scrutinise the evidence of risk to others from both the clinical team and other agencies, before the patient is discharged from detention in hospital, or significant changes are made to the care plan (see paragraph 3.21).

> ## Managing Dangerous People with Severe Personality Disorder: Case Study 'B'
>
> B is currently serving a 3 year prison sentence. He has a history of offending against female strangers and has a low threshold to violence exacerbated by substance abuse. He is emotionally unstable and demonstrates disregard for the feelings of others. He was assessed under the Mental Health Act 1983 as having a psychopathic disorder, but is 'untreatable'. The most recent sentence is for possession of an offensive weapon and agencies are working in partnership to manage his eventual release, since he regularly breaches his licence conditions.
>
> The new arrangements would affect B whilst still in prison. He would undergo a specialist DSPD assessment in a prison assessment facility which would provide a more comprehensive picture of the risk he poses to others and his needs than current assessments carried out under the Mental Health Act 1983. If transfer to hospital was appropriate, the transfer direction would carry a restriction order which would allow him to be conditionally discharged with help and support in the community, required to reside in a specialist rehabilitation hostel if appropriate, and quickly recalled to hospital if necessary. If hospital care was not appropriate, he would be transferred to a suitable Prison Service facility that provides Prison Service regimes and other interventions relating to his identified needs. The statutory duty on health and social services agencies to share information with others where justified will ensure effective risk management when B is eventually discharged/released into the community.

Role of the Tribunal for patients subject to restrictions

4.15 Where the Court has imposed a restriction order, it will be on the basis of a risk assessment which concludes that because of behaviours associated with mental disorder, or for other reasons, the offender poses a significant risk of serious harm to others. The Court will expressly have given the Home Secretary the responsibility to monitor the management of such offenders and to scrutinise the pace of their rehabilitation from the viewpoint of the protection of the public. The Home Secretary will retain the responsibility in this regard that he has had under the 1983 Act. He will remain the primary authority for the discharge of these offenders. Accordingly, for patients subject to restrictions, the role of the new Mental Health Tribunal will be similar to that of the Mental Health Review Tribunal under the 1983 Act. The Tribunal will be required to review the offender's liability to detention in hospital for treatment, and ensure that it remains justified, rather than considering an application for making or renewing a care and treatment order as described in Chapter Three for civil patients.

4.16 Review of detention would be on the basis of whether there was continuing evidence that:

- the patient is suffering from a mental disorder;

- the mental disorder must be of a nature or degree as to warrant specialist care and treatment;

- a plan of care and treatment must be available to address the mental disorder. In cases where the use compulsory powers arises primarily in the patient's own best interests, that plan must be anticipated to be of direct therapeutic benefit to the individual concerned. In cases where compulsory powers are sought primarily because of the risk that the patient poses to others, the plan must be considered necessary either directly to treat the underlying mental disorder or to manage behaviours arising from the disorder.

Role of Parole Board for prisoners serving a life sentence

4.17 The Parole Board will continue to have responsibility for release of a life sentence prisoner who is subject to a hospital direction or is transferred to hospital from prison. Whilst detained under powers in the new legislation, a patient who is subject to a life sentence will be able to apply to the Tribunal for a review of his or her liability to compulsory care and treatment. If a Tribunal decides that the criteria for compulsory care and treatment are no longer met, the patient will be returned to prison. If he or she has served the tariff imposed by the Court, they will be eligible on return to prison to apply to the Parole Board for release.

Discharge of restricted patients from hospital and provisions for recall

4.18 The Tribunal hearing an application from a restricted patient will be able to make a discharge subject to conditions, as in the 1983 Act. If the Tribunal concludes that it is no longer appropriate for the patient to be liable to compulsory care and treatment, it will be required to order absolute discharge.

4.19 The Tribunal might conclude, on the basis of a proposed care plan, that the criteria for continuing liability to care and treatment under compulsory powers are met, but that detention for treatment in hospital is not appropriate. In these circumstances the Tribunal could order discharge from hospital conditional on compliance with the care plan. The issues to be considered by the Tribunal would be similar to those for making a care and treatment order in the community (see paragraphs 3.22, 3.23). Conditions of discharge will include supervision by social and psychiatric supervisors, who will be required to report regularly to the Home Secretary.

4.20 The Home Secretary will retain the power of recall to hospital as in the 1983 Act. The grounds for recall will be that:

- the patient continues to suffer from a mental disorder within the meaning of the new legislation; and,

- the patient is failing to co-operate with the care plan stipulated as a condition of discharge; and/or,

- the patient's continued presence in the community poses a risk of serious harm to others; and/or,

- the patient requires care and treatment that cannot be provided safely or effectively in the community.

4.21 A patient who is subject to conditional discharge will have the right to apply to the Tribunal for review of liability to continuing compulsory care and treatment or liability to compulsory recall under the new legislation. As now, on the basis of evidence from the clinical team and/or independent experts, the Home Secretary or the Tribunal will be able to discharge the patient absolutely from compulsory powers.

4.22 A lawyer with experience of sentencing in the Higher Courts will chair a Mental Health Tribunal hearing an application or reference of a restricted patient. This is essential to preserving the confidence of the sentencing Court in the efficacy of powers for compulsory care and treatment as an alternative to a prison sentence.

Provision of information to victims of mentally disordered offenders

4.23 There was strong support in the responses to the Green Paper, *Reform of the Mental Health Act 1983*[8], for the proposal that more information should be provided to the victims of offenders given a Mental Health Act disposal by the courts rather than a prison sentence.

4.24 The Government is committed to improving the level of service provided to victims generally and in particular to giving proper recognition to the needs of victims of mentally disordered offenders. The new legislation will contain provisions to allow victims of mentally disordered offenders to be given appropriate information about the offender's detention and discharge. Where the Tribunal is considering discharge, we aim to enable victims to make representations to the Tribunal about discharge conditions that relate to contact with them or their family. These provisions will be aimed at providing broader parity of treatment between the victims of mentally disordered offenders and other offenders.

4.25 The provisions will relate to the victims of offenders who have committed serious violent or sexual offences and who are detained in hospital for care and treatment. They will also relate to the victim of an offender who received a prison sentence from the court but has subsequently been transferred to hospital under the new legislation and remains detained in hospital as a civil patient on expiry of his prison sentence.

[8] Reform of the Mental Health Act 1983. Proposals for Consultation CM.4480. TSO.

Chapter Five

Information sharing and risk management

5.1 It is vital for the effective protection of the public that information on patients who are assessed as posing a risk of serious harm to others as a result of their mental disorder is able to be exchanged between those agencies involved in the patient's care and treatment (health and social services), and other relevant agencies, particularly criminal justice agencies.

5.2 The new legislation will include a new statutory duty covering the disclosure of information about patients suffering from mental disorder between health and social services agencies and other agencies (for example, housing and criminal justice agencies), where it can be justified. This will include cases where there is a significant risk of serious harm to others from the patient. Such information will of course be kept confidential by the receiving agencies (except in those limited and specified circumstances where its release is justified, for example, where specific individuals are thought to be at risk of harm from the person concerned and would need to be alerted for their own safety).

5.3 There will also be a duty on health and social services agencies to ensure that appropriate arrangements for storing and exchanging confidential patient information with other agencies are in place. Guidance in the Code of Practice on the new legislation will support the application of the new power and set out general principles that should be followed. (See Part One, paragraph 5.34.)

Good Practice

Risk Assessment, Management and Audit System (RAMAS)

RAMAS is a multi-agency approach to risk assessment and management which was developed in 1994 to specifically address concerns raised by inquiries into homicides by individuals with mental disorder. It aims to:

- ensure that people who pose a risk to themselves or others do not 'fall through the care net';

- ensure that a comprehensive health, social and personal needs assessment is carried out for everyone who comes into contact with services;

- ensure that a clear, accurate, complete risk and care assessment is carried out in order to collate the 'intelligence' through which robust risk and care management and audit may be made;

- to provide a common language for inter-agency communication and collaboration on risk and care;

- facilitate an integrated, co-ordinated, user friendly and positive approach to public safety and individual care;

- facilitate case and workload management through a standardised method which provides evidence-based care, clear, shared goals and good practice.

Contact: Dr Margaret O'Rourke, Consultant Forensic Clinical Psychologist,
Tel: 01483 452754. Website: www.ramas.co.uk

Local arrangements for risk assessment and management in the community of potentially dangerous offenders

5.4 Multi Agency Risk Panels, or Public Protection Panels have been established across the country primarily to satisfy the requirements of the Sex Offender Act 1997, which placed a duty on the police to monitor those offenders who are required to be on the sex offender register. Many panels have subsequently extended their remit to respond to the risks posed by other potentially dangerous offenders in their communities and a range of agencies are now involved in local arrangements, led by police and probation services.

5.5 The Criminal Justice and Court Services Act 2000 amends the Sex Offenders Act 1997 and places a statutory duty on police and probation services to establish arrangements for the assessment and management of risks posed by relevant sexual or violent offenders in the community, and to monitor those arrangements. It also broadens the scope of those subject to these local risk management arrangements to include offenders who have received a hospital order under the Mental Health Act 1983 following conviction for a sexual or violent offence. The provisions are expected to come into force on 1 April 2001.

5.6 Guidance will shortly be issued to responsible authorities on the discharge of their functions under these new statutory provisions. This will be based on a recent review by the Home Office of good practice in risk management arrangements across the country. The guidance will stress the importance of involvement by agencies such as health, social services and housing in support of the police and probation services.

5.7 Provisions for a new statutory duty covering the disclosure of patient information between health and social services agencies and other agencies where it is justified, for example, in the public interest, will support these new risk management arrangements led by the criminal justice system. It is only by effective inter-agency working that the right risk management packages for individuals will be put in place and risk managed in the most effective way.

Chapter Six

Managing high risk individuals – service development

Introduction

6.1 The Government has recognised that in many instances patients who pose (or have posed) a high risk to others are not receiving the most appropriate or effective care and treatment that they need and in some cases, are held in inappropriate levels of security. This section describes a number of changes already underway which are designed to meet these problems. The emphasis is on improving the evidence-base of 'what works' through research and expanding the range of services provided to better meet the needs of all patient groups. This section also sets out in detail the proposed changes to the organisation and delivery of services for the DSPD group over the next three years.

6.2 The clarification and enhancement of the legal provisions which enable the compulsory care and treatment of individuals with mental disorder who pose a risk of serious harm to others, described in Chapter Three, will not reduce the risk to the public on their own. In order effectively to protect the public and safeguard the rights of individual patients, it is essential that robust legal powers are balanced with the delivery of high quality specialist care and treatment, at the right level of security, to meet the needs of individuals and reduce the risk they pose to others.

Developing secure mental health services

Provision of high security psychiatric services

6.3 Section 4 of the NHS Act 1977 was amended by section 41 of the Health Act 1999 to allow high security psychiatric services to be provided by NHS trusts. The aim of this change was to allow the three Special Hospital Authorities (Broadmoor, Ashworth and Rampton) to form new organisations with existing mental health trusts, so that they become providers of high security psychiatric services within an integrated secure and general mental health services trust.

6.4 Plans for Broadmoor and Rampton Hospital Authorities to integrate with other NHS trusts providing a wider range of mental health services are already well advanced. Broadmoor Hospital Authority will be dissolved on 31 March 2001, with a new West London Mental Health NHS Trust, incorporating Broadmoor Hospital and Ealing, Hammersmith and Fulham Mental Health Trust, becoming operational on 1 April 2001. Rampton Hospital Authority will also be dissolved on 31 March 2001, with a new Nottinghamshire Healthcare NHS Trust, incorporating Rampton Hospital and the medium secure services within Trent Region, becoming operational on 1 April 2001.

6.5 The integration arrangements for Ashworth Hospital Authority are linked to the wider development of secure psychiatric services in the North West. In this respect, formal consultation has begun on the creation of a new Mersey Mental Health Trust, which is expected to be established from April 2001. The proposal being consulted upon envisages that the mental illness service provided by Ashworth Hospital will form part of the new trust at a later date. Options for the other services currently provided by Ashworth Hospital Authority are currently being considered.

6.6 The high security hospitals' professional and geographical isolation has undoubtedly been at the root of many of the difficulties they have experienced. The integration of each of the hospitals into NHS trusts providing a wider range of mental health services will considerably alleviate the isolation problem, and there are already indications that recruitment difficulties are improving. The distinction between high and medium secure services will be maintained by providing the services on separate sites but with the advantage of having a Trust Board which can take an overview of the provision of the whole range of services.

6.7 We are confident that the new investment in the high security hospitals, and the linked modernisation and mainstreaming of the hospitals, will achieve our twin objectives of securing the safety of the public, staff and patients whilst offering a high quality service to people who genuinely require care and treatment in a high security setting.

Commissioning secure mental health services

6.8 Regional Specialised Commissioning Groups, which this year took on full responsibility for the commissioning of high and medium secure psychiatric services, are providing a more focused mechanism for identifying the needs of their population and developing integrated local services. Devolution of the funding for high security services from the High Security Psychiatric Services Commissioning Team within the NHS Executive to Health Authorities has removed the perverse financial incentive for health authorities to take patients back once they no longer require conditions of high security, and will facilitate the movement of patients into the level of security which they genuinely need.

6.9 The following will be essential components of the new commissioning arrangements:

- the formulation of a regional strategy agreed by all the key stakeholders. This will encompass robust assessment of patient needs, definitions of patient categories and admission criteria, and staffing and service development requirements for the local population of patients needing all levels of secure services;

- the involvement and commitment of providers (managers and clinicians) in the development of a strategic plan, the commissioning process and the co-ordination of service development;

- the involvement of local authorities, criminal justice agencies, social care, voluntary agencies, the Prison Service, and user representatives in the co-ordination of strategic planning and commissioning;

- management of the interface between the commissioning arrangements for high and medium security services and the commissioning of general mental health services;

- management of local commissioning in the context of the national priorities for provision of high and medium secure services, including the provision of low volume specialist secure services (for example for people with learning disabilities, women and hearing impaired patients);

- national oversight of the process.

Review of security at the high security hospitals and reprovision of medium security services

6.10 In 1999, the Department of Health commissioned a review of security at the high security hospitals by a team led by Sir Richard Tilt, the former Director General of the Prison Service. Sir Richard's report,[9] published earlier this year, made a number of recommendations for improvements to the perimeter and internal security of the hospitals, all of which we have accepted. We have made the necessary funding available and work is currently under way to implement those recommendations.

6.11 The Government has commissioned a review of medium security provision and forensic networks of care, which will identify gaps in capacity. The review will also encompass a survey of all types of secure beds, and the results will be shared with the appropriate agencies.

6.12 The Government has made an extra £25 million of recurrent revenue funding available, phased in over a three year period, specifically to address the problem of moving out patients when they no longer require treatment in conditions of high security. Significant capital funding is also being made available for this purpose over the three years 2001/04. The needs assessment work currently being undertaken will help inform the use of this funding, and women patients will be given high priority.

Developing secure women's services

6.13 The Department of Health commissioned work, supported by an expert group chaired by Dame Rennie Fritchie[10], to look at strategic issues around women in the high security hospitals. The report of this group was published in March 1999.

6.14 This report is forming the basis of the development of a strategy, linked to additional funding, to ensure that priority is given to the discharge and movement out of the high secure hospitals of women patients who have been identified as not requiring the physical security that the three hospitals provide. The ultimate aim will be to provide safe, appropriate, and secure services that meet the needs of women patients. The strategy should be complete within 12 months.

6.15 However, it is likely that there will remain a very small number of women who present a high risk to the safety of others and who will continue to require a high level of physical security. The longer term needs of these women will be considered further by the National Oversight Group in policy and strategic developments around implementation of Sir Richard Tilt's report, and will also form part of policy considerations between the Department of Health and the Home Office around services for women who are DSPD. Consideration will be given to creating separate dedicated facilities for the small number of women who require high secure care.

Forensic child and adolescent mental health services

6.16 The Government recognises that action is required to bring fragmented and variable local services for children and adolescents with mental health problems up to an acceptable standard. Joint national targets for child and adolescent mental health services (CAMHS) for health and social care were introduced for the first time under the National Priorities Guidance 1999-2002, backed by additional investment from the NHS Modernisation Fund and the Mental Health Grant to local authorities.

[9] Report of the Review of Security at the High Security Hospitals Department of Health. May 2000.

[10] Secure Futures for Women: Making a Difference. March 1999. Available from the Department of Health.

6.17 We are working on the development of a strategy for forensic CAMHS. The intention is that this will cover all levels of need and service provision, including in-patient services and specialist community outreach teams. The need for additional CAMHS forensic secure units will be considered as part of our development strategy.

Prison mental health services

6.18 The Government recognises the need for, and is committed to delivering, reform of the health care services to prisoners, including young offenders. The report of a joint Prison Service/NHS Executive Working Group on the *Future Organisation of Prison Health Care*[11], made a range of recommendations about how improvements should be taken forward on the basis of partnership between the Prison Service and the NHS including, in particular, meeting the needs of prisoners with mental health problems.

6.19 The Government has accepted the Report's recommendations and implementation has started in a number of areas. In particular:

- two new joint units – a Policy Unit and a Task Force – have been established to lead and co-ordinate the reform programme. The units, located in the Department of Health, came into being on 1 April 2000;

- work has also started at a local level, with prisons, young offender institutions and health authorities reviewing jointly the health needs of the local prisoner population. The aim is to develop local improvement plans to shape and focus local health services both inside and outside prison, so that the needs of prisoners and their throughcare are better met.

6.20 *The NHS Plan* recognises the high prevalence of mental health problems among the prison population. For example, recent surveys[12] show that 9 out of 10 adult prisoners have one or more problems related to psychosis, neurosis, personality disorder and drug or alcohol abuse. Around 5000 prisoners at any one time are estimated to have a serious mental health problem requiring an active intervention. *The NHS Plan*, in keeping with recommendations of the *Report on the Future Organisation of Prison Health Care*, commits to the provisions of an extra 300 NHS staff to provide mental health in-reach services to prisoners, so that their mental health needs are met, and that they do not leave prison without a care plan.

6.21 The in-reach of multi-disciplinary community mental health teams can be expected greatly to improve the standards of care and treatment of mentally disordered prisoners, including those needing transfer to hospital and to facilitate continuity of care, when persons are received into custody, on transfer to hospital and back, and on release back to the community. Appropriately targeted funds will be made available to health authorities so that mental health services may reach in those prisons with mentally disordered offenders.

6.22 As part of the development of the in-reach of services, existing protocols will be reviewed and revised so that transparent referral and transfer arrangements are in place for those prisoners who need in-patient treatment for mental disorder in hospital or in a DSPD treatment centre. At present around 750 prisoners are transferred to hospital as restricted patients under the Mental Health Act 1983 each year. At any one time there will be a number of prisoner-patients waiting either to be assessed or transferred to hospital, and who are at present sometimes held in unsuitable conditions. The

[11] The Future Organisation of Prison Health Care. Reports by the Joint Prison Service and NHS Executive Working Group. March 1999.

[12] Psychiatric Morbidity among prisoners in England and Wales. Office for National Statistics. 1998.

restructuring of the high security psychiatric service, improvements to the organisation of prison health services and in-reach of NHS specialist care will tackle the needs of a group of prisoner-patients who, though they may periodically need the support of a hospital environment, also need to receive more appropriate support and therapeutic intervention whilst in prison.

Developing specialist services for those who are dangerous and severely personality disordered

Introduction

6.23 The challenges posed by those who are DSPD cannot be solved by new legislative powers alone. Before new powers can be applied safely and ethically to those who are DSPD, new specialist assessment and treatment services must also be developed. In practice, many of those who are DSPD cannot safely be managed within mainstream high security psychiatric wards, even if there were capacity to accommodate them in existing services. More fundamentally, in common with many respondents to the consultation exercise and the Home Affairs Select Committee, the Government believes that where individuals are detained as a result of their mental disorder, they must be held in a therapeutic environment which is designed to address their needs effectively. This is not just a matter of new places – important though that is – but also properly trained staff, new approaches to assessment and treatment and a rigorous programme of research and evaluation. We believe that it is important to develop capacity in both the Prison Service and the NHS because, however services for this group are configured in the future, they will need to draw on the skills and expertise of both services. However, this service development phase is also an important opportunity to pilot new approaches to assessment and treatment and to develop a 'what works' evidence-base before taking final decisions about the structure of any new services and how the new powers be applied. The pilot period will also inform decisions about the precise kind of services required, the settings which are most appropriate, and how quickly services would need to be expanded. An important aspect of this work will also be to look at how best to provide specialist services for women who are DSPD.

6.24 The following sections set out our strategy for service development. All the initiatives in this section are being managed under the joint Home Office, Department of Health, Prison Service Programme that has already been described at paragraph 2.16.

New capacity

6.25 The Government has already announced an ambitious programme of service development in the Prison Service and the NHS. The first pilot assessment centre at HMP Whitemoor opened in September and Rampton High Security Hospital has now started piloting the assessment process on its current population of male personality disordered patients. Over the next three years, new approaches to assessment and treatment will be piloted and systematically evaluated in new facilities in both services. The results of this comprehensive programme will feed into decisions about further service development beyond the forthcoming Spending Review period.

Specialist DSPD places within the NHS

6.26 The NHS plan, published in July, announced the expansion of provision of specialist services for DSPD individuals over the next three years. £56m has been allocated to provide:

- 140 additional specialist secure places for the DSPD group by April 2004;

- 75 specialist rehabilitation hostel places by April 2004 to enable those personality disordered patients assessed as safe to be discharged into the community to move out of secure facilities more quickly and receive specialist help and support in the community.

Specialist DSPD facilities within the Prison Service

6.27 In the Prison Service, £70m has been allocated to provide:

- 80 refurbished places – to be fully operational by October 2001

- 100 places in newly built units to open in April 2003

6.28 Because we anticipate that far fewer women will be assessed as being DSPD than men, these facilities are for men only. Decisions on how best to pilot new approaches and provide services for women, will follow on from a detailed study over the next twelve months into their numbers and characteristics within existing services and consideration of how best new approaches to assessment and treatment can be developed and validated for use with women.

Towards a new 'whole system' service approach

6.29 As these new facilities come on stream they will be used to pilot new approaches to the assessment and treatment of those who are DSPD. Within the Prison Service, the pilot services will be used under present legislative powers for sentenced prisoners on a voluntary basis. Within the NHS, pilot sites will be used under current Mental Health Act powers from the beginning. However, not only will these pilots sites be used for the testing out and evaluation of new approaches, they will also provide the core of new services following the implementation of new mental health legislation. These pilot sites could also provide the core of a new 'third service' if, following a period of evaluation and review, the Government decides to proceed with that option. Although the Government has not yet decided whether new dedicated facilities will be required for women, any future powers and any organisational structures based in statute must apply equally to men and women.

6.30 This service development period also means that as new powers come into force the facilities are already in place to allow them to be used. Within the NHS, this transition should be relatively straightforward since any new facilities will already have been operating under mental health legislation. Within the Prison Service, the situation will be more complex because there will need to be a transition from voluntary pilot projects to new statutory arrangements. The Prison Service DSPD assessment facilities will be used to carry out assessments of sentenced prisoners, using the new power of the Home Secretary to direct a prisoner to undergo a specialist mental health assessment (see paragraph 4.11). Where following an assessment, no order is made under the Mental Health Act to transfer the prisoner to an NHS DSPD facility, the prisoner may, if appropriate, be transferred to a suitable Prison Service facility that provides prison service regimes and other interventions relating to the prisoner's identified needs.

Managing DSPD individuals across the Prison Service and the NHS

6.31 However, the Government is determined that any new capacity developed in existing services should not perpetuate a fragmented approach to the management of this group. New services will therefore be developed in a holistic way with partnership arrangements between new settings a fundamental prerequisite both for the identification of new sites and their day to day running. This will ensure that new approaches can consciously draw on the best in existing provision and that common standards are consistently applied in both settings. Practitioners will therefore be encouraged to work across the interface between the prison service and the NHS. For example, close links have already been developed between the Whitemoor Prison and Rampton Hospital pilots involving, for example, staff exchange.

6.32 Moving individuals between the two services according to their needs, and therefore altering the powers under which they are held, will require significant oversight especially in the early days. Individuals being assessed and those who are subsequently detained under powers in new mental health legislation will be detained in an appropriate therapeutic environment.

6.33 Offenders serving a prison sentence who require assessment for DSPD will be assessed in specialist DSPD assessment centres within the prison service. On the basis of the findings of such assessments it will be open to the Home Secretary to make a direction to transfer an offender to hospital if such a transfer is considered by him to be appropriate.

6.34 Offenders before the Courts may be assessed in a hospital whilst on remand. Courts will take into account the findings of such assessments in making sentencing decisions. If an offender is assessed as being DSPD it will be open to the Court to pass a prison sentence combined with a hospital direction or to make a disposal under new mental health legislation. In either case, the offender will be detained in a secure hospital.

6.35 Decisions on more detailed service planning will follow on from the evidence of the pilot projects as more information becomes available about the numbers and characteristics of those who are DSPD. But it is reasonable to anticipate that in the early days there may be problems matching supply to demand in different parts of the country, something that will be particularly important in planning provision for screening and full DSPD assessment.

6.36 Therefore, as part of the DSPD programme of work, before new legislation is implemented a small project team – including operational staff from the Prison Service and NHS – will be established. The team will work alongside existing management structures to:

- manage the transitional process from the pilot process to the application of new powers;

- manage the demand for screening assessments for individuals in the community in the early years of service development and places in the DSPD assessment centres in both prison and NHS;

- manage demand for places in DSPD treatment facilities in both the NHS and the prison service, given the restrictions on where some individuals can be held;

- act as a focal point for clinicians and staff working in both prison service and hospital facilities to ensure that all future decisions about service developments at a local level are taken within the context of the overall pilot and research programme;

- maintain links with other personality disorder services in the NHS and specialist regimes in the prison service eg HMP Grendon – to assist in the management of those individuals assessed as having a personality disorder but who fall below the criteria for entry into the specialist DSPD service.

6.37 In due course, depending on the outcomes of the first phase of the pilot programme, such a central coordinating unit could take on responsibility for the commissioning of specialist DSPD places in both the Prison Service and the NHS, as a further step in bringing the two services more closely together.

The assessment process

6.38 The consultation paper outlined the need for a systematic approach to the determination of whether an individual had a severe personality disorder and the level of risk posed to others. In addition, it would assess any treatment needs, and lead to a plan of care and management that took account of public safety and the full range interventions required. As part of the consultation process (see paragraph 2.9), a group chaired by Dr David Thornton (Head of the Offending Behaviour Programme Unit, Prison Service) developed the outline of such a process which has been further worked up and is now being piloted at Whitemoor Prison and Rampton Hospital. The process falls into two parts: the screening assessment and the full DSPD assessment.

The screening assessment

6.39 The screening assessment will take place in the Prison Service for those detained in prison, and in the NHS for those detained under mental health legislation or those living in the community. The purpose of the screening assessment is to establish whether there is sufficient evidence of someone being DSPD to justify a longer-term intensive assessment, and to establish whether the individual is sufficiently robust to undergo the full assessment.

6.40 As part of the screening assessment, an individual's history will be considered and there will be an interview with clinical staff to assess suitability and to screen out more immediate mental health or other needs e.g. treatment for substance misuse. The screening assessment will be evaluated alongside the full DSPD assessment.

6.41 In the early days, specialist teams will be trained in the screening process at the pilot sites. Following the implementation of the new legislation, regional teams will need to be established to provide access to screening assessments throughout the country.

The specialist DSPD assessment

6.42 The full specialist DSPD assessment will take place at a specialist assessment centre located in either the Prison Service high security estate, or a high security hospital. As presently designed, the assessment process lasts 12 weeks but this will be reviewed as part of the evaluation of the pilot projects.

6.43 As with the screening assessment, a multi-disciplinary team will conduct the assessment. The assessment process will include a range of risk assessments, and psychiatric, psychological, as well as behavioural and social observation. At the end of the process a case conference will identify whether the individual has a severe personality disorder, whether his or her level of risk is sufficiently high to justify being managed in a secure DSPD treatment setting, and whether the risk presented is linked to the personality disorder. It will also identify any specific treatment needs. The findings will be set out in a report which will cover the results of individual tools and instruments used and contain the actuarial and clinical data to substantiate its conclusions. These reports will be available to judges in informing sentencing decisions for those before the Courts, and to Mental Health Tribunals as part of civil proceedings for detention under new mental health legislation.

6.44 A psychiatrist will be a core member of any assessment team so that if either during, or as a result of, the assessment a person displays symptoms of a mental illness, appropriate services can quickly be identified. There will also be individuals who, after assessment, are found to pose a high risk to others, but who are not personality disordered. In the case of individuals who have been assessed on remand at the order of a Court, information from the assessment process may still be helpful to the Court when considering sentencing, the Prison Service in sentence planning and the Probation Service in supervising offenders in the community. Where the individual is not currently before the courts, information on the risk they pose will be used by local risk management panels to put in place a plan to manage the risk the individual poses (see paragraphs 5.4-5.6).

Assessment of women who may be DSPD

6.45 The DSPD assessment process being piloted at HMP Whitemoor and Rampton Hospital applies to men only. However, new legislative powers will apply equally to men and women and this will need to be supported by the provision of appropriate services. A separate project has therefore been established to identify and provide for the needs of women including plans for separate pilots of the assessment process and new approaches to treatment (see paragraphs 6.68 and 6.69).

Assessment of dangerousness and personality disorder in young people

6.46 Assessment of dangerousness in young people presents an even greater challenge than adults given the developmental factors involved. It is not currently known how to accurately identify those in adolescence who will be assessed as falling into the DSPD group once they reach adulthood (see paragraph 6.71).

6.47 Young people may be detained under the Mental Health Act for mental disorder or under section 25 of the Children Act, if they meet the relevant criteria defined in the Acts. Some are detained in young offenders institutions following conviction for a criminal offence. Further work will be required to address the legal transitions and the interface issues between services for young people and adult DSPD services to ensure that mechanisms are put in place to provide ongoing care and treatment for such young people once they reach 18 years. In a very small number of such cases it may be necessary to arrange for immediate assessment for compulsory care and treatment in a specialist adult DSPD service under mental health legislation.

Evaluation

6.48 Rigorous, independent analysis of the DSPD assessment process will be a key part of the service development process and a contract for the evaluation of the process has now been let. The evaluation will examine whether the assessment process:

- is valid, reliable and user friendly (including the impact on staff);

- is predictive of re-offending, quality of life, social integration, overall better functioning;

- identifies co-existing mental illness, learning disability, substance misuse, physical ill-health;

- is non-discriminatory, fair, culturally sensitive and takes account of the needs of those from ethnic minorities;

- identifies wider treatment needs e.g. health, social, educational, occupational and criminogenic.

Treatment

6.49 The DSPD assessment will provide information not only to inform the decisions of the courts and Mental Health Tribunals, but also to identify the care and treatment needs of the individuals concerned. It will be a requirement of any compulsory care and treatment order under the new legislation that, where compulsory powers are sought primarily because of the risk that the patient poses to others, a care plan is available that is considered necessary either directly to treat the underlying mental disorder, or to manage behaviours arising from mental disorder. Therefore new capacity for care and treatment and the development of new approaches is a fundamental part of the Government's service development strategy.

Therapeutic interventions

6.50 DSPD is a working definition rather than a single clinical diagnosis (see paragraph 2.18). We anticipate that any DSPD population will include a number of sub-groups i.e. individuals who pose a high risk to others as a result of a variety of different personality disorders. A number of therapies and approaches have been shown to be effective with particular groups and it is important to build on these in developing a comprehensive range of treatments. It will also be important to ensure that treatment regimes are sensitive to the needs of those from ethnic minorities. As part of the service development process, there will be two new treatment pilots within the Prison Service. The first of these at Whitemoor Prison will open in October 2001 and provide two new units each of 25 places. Within the NHS, new units for treating those who are DSPD will also be established.

6.51 Initially these pilots will be based on the best of current knowledge drawing on both the experience of existing NHS personality disorder services and work in the Prison Service. We will also be drawing on international practice and research. However, we will be considering whether recent innovative approaches can also be incorporated within the overall programme for example:

- programmes being developed in the Prison Service for those with "high Hare scores", previously found to be resistant to conventional approaches;

- Dialectical Behaviour Therapy;

- therapeutic regimes such as that at HMP Grendon;

- other cognitive behavioural therapies; and,

- community therapeutic programmes.

6.52 It is envisaged that any final treatment programme will be tailored to the individual patient. It is possible that there might be a core treatment programme for most of those who are DSPD, but most therapeutic interventions will be selected from a wider menu to meet individual treatment needs.

6.53 However, as the Royal College of Psychiatrists' Report on Offenders with Personality Disorder[13] concluded, there is a need to define and refine current treatment goals for offenders with personality disorder and to undertake long term randomised trials with long-term follow up. The treatment approaches that are to be provided at the pilot sites will be evaluated in terms of a range of outcomes including levels of change in psychological state and reconviction. Where programmes have been shown to work they will be re-evaluated at regular intervals to monitor outcomes to check that standards have been maintained. The design of the evaluations will be robust. The strongest design for an evaluation is random allocation of subjects and this will be considered and chosen if possible (subject to ethical considerations).

6.54 At present little is known about effective treatment for female offenders suffering from personality disorder and who pose a risk to others. There is some evidence to suggest that therapeutic communities, cognitive-behavioural and dialectical behavioural therapies may be effective in treating some individuals. Work is currently underway to map out the therapeutic interventions currently available or suitable for high risk women in Prison and NHS settings. We intend to draw on this mapping exercise in devising and piloting a range of treatment interventions for women identified as DSPD.

[13] The Royal College of Psychiatrists Council Report CR 71 – Offenders with Personality Disorder.

Good Practice

Rampton High Security Hospital Personality Disorder Service

The Personality Disorder Service was established in 1994 to provide a dedicated specialist service for mentally disordered offenders with severe personality disorder who require high security hospital care. The primary goal of service is to reduce the level of risk the individual presents to others through their dysfunctional lifestyle so that they are able to move towards living in less secure conditions.

A therapeutic milieu is offered within a structured living environment which focuses mainly on addressing outstanding clinical needs by modelling and promoting appropriate interpersonal interactions. This is done through providing a series of structured, mainly cognitive behavioural groups. All groups are supplemented by intensive individual nursing and psychology interventions.

A personality disorder beacon service.
Contact through the NHS beacon team. Tel: 01730 235018
email: nhsbeacons@statusmeetings.co.uk

Good Practice

East Midlands Centre for Mental Health – Medium secure facility for personality disordered offenders

Arnold Lodge contains a 10-bedded medium security unit for men with personality disorder and a history of serious offending. A 15-month programme is provided which is designed to ameliorate skills deficits of offenders and examine whether the skills acquired are used. There is a strong community focus, and multi-agency working with referring and receiving agencies. 70% of admissions come from the prison service.

A personality disorder beacon service.
Contact through the NHS beacon team.
Tel: 01730 235018 email: nhsbeacons@statusmeetings.co.uk

Good Practice

HMP Grendon – Therapeutic community

Grendon Prison consists of five autonomous therapeutic communities which provide a rigorous treatment programme for those with severe personality disorder who are serving a long sentence. The approach has been demonstrated to dramatically reduce the re-conviction rates of life-sentenced prisoners who stay 18 months or more in Grendon.

A personality disorder beacon service.
Contact through the NHS beacon team. Tel: 01730 235018
email: nhsbeacons@statusmeetings.co.uk

Developing effective community services

Discharge and rehabilitation

6.55 Those who are DSPD need to be detained in an effective therapeutic environment both in order to ensure that they are managed safely and ethically but also to enable them to work towards successful re-integration into the community. However, when individuals are assessed as safe to be released or discharged into the community, it is likely that treatments delivered in a secure setting will need to be 'topped up' in the community. Some may also require some form of supported hostel accommodation to help them to make the transition to life in the community.

New provision for community rehabilitation hostels

6.56 There is a recognised lack of suitable community services into which those individuals with personality disorder who are currently in the high security hospitals, and who have been assessed as no longer presenting a high risk to others, can be moved. The NHS Plan announced the provision, by 2004, of 75 specialist rehabilitation hostel places which will enable those SPD patients being discharged into the community to move out of secure facilities more quickly and receive specialist help and support in the community.

Community supervision

6.57 Community supervision will also be important in managing the process of discharge. The Government's commitment to a 'joined-up' service approach extends into the community and we will be working with the Probation Service and health and social services to ensure that expertise is shared and that, as far as possible, common standards are developed irrespective of which service is responsible for statutory supervision on release or discharge into the community. In particular, the Probation Service already has considerable expertise in managing risk and in rehabilitating offenders with severe personality disorder and it will be essential that health and social services work closely with the probation service and build on this knowledge base.

Secondary prevention – preventing future dangerousness

6.58 A multi-disciplinary project team involving representatives from the police, probation and health and social services has been working closely with the range of services and agencies that come into contact with people with personality disorder, to identify the difficulties currently experienced in managing this group of people in the community and any gaps in service provision, and to highlight effective models of multi-disciplinary working. The findings of this work will be made available shortly and will used by the Department of Health and the Home Office to facilitate further service development and effective models of multi-disciplinary working in this area. This work includes effective provision for those being discharged from secure care, and services for those young adults who may develop high risk behaviour and require detention in hospital if they do not received appropriate interventions at an early stage.

Improving local risk management arrangements

6.59 Multi Agency Risk Panels (see paragraphs 5.4 – 5.6) will have a significant role to play in managing the risk posed by dangerous people with severe personality disorder both before and after detention in hospital. They are well placed to monitor the risk posed by individuals in the community and to coordinate agencies' efforts to reduce that risk. Where risk can no longer be effectively managed in the community, they will be able to refer an individual for assessment under new mental health legislation.

Staffing issues

6.60 The provision of new staff, new skills and new ways of working is an important part of our service development strategy. The Human Resources and Training Project has been established to identify and provide for this and to make recommendations about how best and how quickly services can be developed beyond the initial pilot period. The project will work closely with those responsible for human resources in existing services to ensure that any new services are not developed at their expense and that new services are not isolated from mainstream mental health services and criminal justice services.

6.61 Each of the pilot sites will employ a multi-disciplinary workforce. Although in the Prison Service, the majority of the staff will be Prison Officers and in the NHS the majority will be nursing staff, both will also include members of other professions including psychologists, psychiatrists, occupational therapists, probation officers and social workers.

6.62 The pilot site teams will also receive comprehensive specialist training and preparation, in addition to their core skills and knowledge, for working with this group. This will involve the development of team based skills and competency training programmes, and supervision skills training for managers. Recruitment and retention plans will also be developed to help address the difficulties and isolation that staff working with dangerous and severely personality disordered individuals often feel. It will also be important to ensure that new services do not become isolated from mainstream mental health and prison services and career pathways will need to enable staff to enter and leave DSPD services at different points in their careers. These plans will incorporate race equality issues both because of the Government's fundamental commitment to equality of opportunity and because an ethnically and culturally diverse workforce is needed if new services are to be fair, non-discriminatory and culturally sensitive.

6.63 Finally, strong leadership for staff working with DSPD individuals is vital. Training programmes for those who will be managing service delivery will be developed and there will be staff support and supervision training.

Research and international comparisons

6.64 An essential component of the DSPD service development strategy is to increase the evidence base. Findings from previous research studies both nationally and internationally have indicated potentially beneficial interventions for the DSPD group, but the results have limited value (Stein and Brown 1991[14],Davidson and Tyrer 1996[15], Linehan 1993[16]). This is because of the methodology used, the way in which samples have been defined, because follow up has always been relatively short or because the interventions themselves have not yet been evaluated on the higher risk groups with personality disorder. These are factors, which along with previous under funding, have led to a low evidence base and problems in achieving a professional consensus about service development models (Royal College of Psychiatrists 1999[17], Cope 1993[18], Dolan and Coid 1993[19]). This is the global position in respect of those countries where such services are being developed.

6.65 The service development and pilot approach that we have adopted incorporates a rigorous research programme. An essential component of this is the development and maintenance of international links to share knowledge, to learn from each other, and to carry out research together. Of the countries where we already have good links, for example The Netherlands and Canada, considerable thought is being given to taking forward similar evaluative work in respect of their own services. To this end, we are taking a new and innovative approach in establishing formal working links, building on existing international links, for example, the Anglo Dutch Accord (SHSA 1995[20]).

6.66 Rigorous evaluation will be a fundamental part of the development of new services. The Government is determined that the future expansion of services and decisions about how best to structure and manage services for this group will be based on an evolving evidence-base. This will in part be provided by the evaluation of the pilot projects. But a wider research programme alongside this work is needed to fill other gaps in current knowledge. Substantial resources have been allocated to fund a comprehensive research programme – £2m in 2001/02 and comparable sums in the following two years. In addition to evaluating the pilot projects, the research programme will include:

- work to refine the numbers and characteristics of people who are DSPD;

- work to identify the causes of personality disorder in order to develop therapeutic interventions among those at risk of developing DSPD;

- cohort studies to assess the validity of the assessment process in predicting reconviction and aim to identify the risk factors associated with re-offending in this group;

- a long-term follow-up study of offenders with personality disorder in the community to assess the criminogenic needs of this group; and,

- work to ensure that every aspect of service development is non-discriminatory and culturally sensitive to the needs of those from ethnic minorities.

[14] Stein,E.and Brown,J.D (1991) Group therapy in a forensic setting. Canadian Journal of Psychiatry, **36**, 718-722.

[15] Davidson,K. and Tyrer,P. (1996) Cognitive therapy for antisocial and borderline personality disorder:single case study series. British Journal of Clinical Psychology, **35**, 413-429.

[16] Linehan,M.M. (1993) Cognitive Behavioral Treatment of Borderline Personality Disorder. The Guilford Press.

[17] The Royal College of Psychiatrists (1999) Offenders with Personality Disorder. Council Report CR 71. Gaskell.

[18] Cope,R.(1993) A survey of forensic psychiatrists views on psychopathic disorder.Journal of Forensic Psychiatry, **4**, 215-235.

[19] Dolan,B. and Coid,J. (1993)Psychopathic and Antisocial Personality Disorders: Treatment and Research Issues. London: Gaskell.

[20] Special Hospitals Service Authority.(1995) Understanding the Enigma. Summary of the Anglo-Dutch Conference on Personality Disorder and Offending.Special Hospitals Service Authority,

6.67 This research agenda has been agreed by an expert group of academics, clinicians and practitioners[21]. This expert group will monitor progress and will quality assure projects within the programme. The highest quality standards will apply and, where possible, research reports will be published and peer reviewed.

Services for women who are dangerous and severely personality disordered

6.68 A separate Women's Services Project has been established in order to give special attention to the needs of women who might be identified as DSPD. This is not intended to imply that new powers will apply any differently to women but rather to mainstream consideration of women's issues within the whole programme of service development. The basic principle underpinning this work is that the criteria that determine identification as DSPD should be the same for men and women. In practice, this means that:

- the level of risk posed must be comparable between men and women DSPDs, although the factors that give rise to the risk, and the ways in which that risk may be demonstrated may differ (e.g. in men: violent sexual acts, in women: life threatening arson);

- the tools used for assessment should be validated for use with men and women;

- the assessment process should be gender aware but not gender biased. For example, it should not deliberately exclude from the identification of DSPD factors that are unusual in men, but more prevalent in women, and are good indicators of high risk;

- treatment programmes for all DSPDs will need to be individually designed. There will be no 'off the shelf' set of interventions, but it likely that there will be a common 'pool' of interventions;

- the range of treatment programmes suitable for use with women may differ from the range available for men, but all will be designed to address the risk posed.

6.69 The Women's Services Project will therefore work alongside other projects to ensure that the needs of women who are DSPD are identified and that specialist services are developed accordingly.

Prevention strategies

6.70 Annex E of the consultation paper outlined a number of Government initiatives being taken forward across a wide range of Government departments and agencies which will help to reduce the numbers of children and adolescents who become severely personality disordered and dangerous by intervening with those children most at risk of developing personality disorder.

[21] The Research and Development Advisory Group of the DSPD Programme.

Primary prevention

6.71 Building on these initiatives, work on primary prevention will be an important part of the DSPD Research Programme. As a first step in developing a strategy to increase our knowledge of the specific causative and protective factors involved in the development of severe anti-social personality disorders, and what interventions are effective in childhood and adolescence in preventing severe personality disorder, the Department of Health and the Home Office commissioned the Policy Research Bureau to conduct a literature review of current knowledge about childhood risk factors for the development of severe personality disorder, and possible interventions. The report is due to be published early in the New Year and will help to inform future research and policy development. This work will be taken forward as part of the Research Strategy.

Conclusion

6.72 Many respondents to the DSPD consultation paper, commented on the need for new investment to develop new capacity, new approaches and the need to develop a strong research base for the future. This programme of work represents a substantial new investment of almost £126m over the next three years. It provides a unique opportunity to address the challenges posed by this group. Our approach is a pragmatic one. Public protection requires that the full range of new powers should be available as soon as possible and that specialist services should be available to allow those powers to be used. But decisions on the further development of those services, the speed of build-up, and their final organisational structure will depend on the expanding knowledge base that this investment will secure.

Glossary of terms

Advanced agreements

An advance agreement sets out a patient's instructions concerning his or her care or treatment. It will usually be made out when the patient has proper ability to make such decisions and is intended to be used to influence treatment when his or her judgment is impaired by their mental disorder. Health professionals are not bound to follow such instructions if they conflict with their professional judgment about the most appropriate form of care and treatment, but they should give them serious consideration.

Care and treatment order

The care and treatment order will authorise the care and treatment specified in a care plan recommended by the clinical team. The order will be made by the Mental Health Tribunal.

Care plan

A comprehensive care plan is prepared by a patient's clinical team following a detailed assessment of the patient's needs carried out in accordance with the Care Programme Approach and the corresponding guidance in Wales. The written care plan will address the patient's identified health and social needs.

Care Programme Approach (CPA)

The CPA provides a framework for care co-ordination of service users under specialist mental health services. The main elements are a care co-ordinator, a written care plan, and at the higher level, regular reviews by the multi-disciplinary health team and integration with the social services care management.

Carers

Professional carers, relatives or friends who look after individuals who are mentally disordered. This will normally be the main carer or carers.

Civil powers

Legal powers of compulsory care and treatment authorised by the Mental Health Tribunal in civil proceedings.

Clinical supervisor

The consultant with lead responsibility for the care of a patient with a mental disorder. Normally a consultant psychiatrist, but may also include a consultant psychologist. The clinical supervisor replaces the current "Responsible Medical Officer".

Clinical team

A multi-disciplinary team, under the leadership of the clinical supervisor, which is responsible for the assessment, care and treatment and supervision of patients.

Code of Practice

A statutory Code of Practice will provide guidance on the operation of the new legislation, and will cover the key areas of good practice. It will be an important source of information for practitioners, patients and their advisers.

Cognitive Behavioural Therapy (CBT)

A form of psychological treatment based on learning theory principles used mostly in depression but increasingly shown to be a useful component of treatment in schizophrenia and some personality disorder. CBT involves improving thinking and social skills by teaching strategies to apply to deal with problems and people more effectively.

Commission for Health Improvement

CHI was set up under the Health Act 1999 to inspect all NHS organisations in a rolling programme to help drive up standards and the quality of care, and began work in April 2000. CHI is the first ever independent, external body to scrutinise standards in the NHS. CHI also has a developmental role in helping the NHS to address weaknesses through providing advice and spreading good practice more quickly and effectively than before.

Commission for Mental Health

The Mental Health Act Commission will be replaced by a new Commission for Mental Health which will look after the interests of people who are subject to the provisions of the new legislation.

Compulsory powers

The legal powers of compulsion which empower the clinical supervisor to provide care and treatment for a mental disorder in the absence of a patient's consent.

Conditional discharge

When a restricted patient is discharged from hospital subject to specified conditions and liability to be recalled to hospital by the Home Secretary.

Criminal justice disposal

A period of imprisonment or a community punishment imposed by a Court.

Criminal justice system

All the agencies responsible for the detection and prosecution of breaches of the criminal law and for the execution of the sentences of Courts. These include the police, the Crown Prosecution Service, the Courts and the probation and prison services.

Dialectical behavioural therapy

A specific type of cognitive behavioural therapy which includes skills training and exposure to emotional cues, found to be particularly effective in treating those with self-harming behaviour. It is delivered according to a manual to ensure adherence to effective interventions.

Discharge

A patient will be discharged from compulsory care and treatment under the new legislation when the conditions for continued use of compulsory powers are no longer met. Discharge from compulsory care and treatment does not mean that a patient will not need continuing care but in many cases care and treatment will continue without the use of compulsory powers.

Emergency powers

Powers to detain a patient pending a preliminary examination to determine whether the use of compulsory powers is appropriate.

Expert panel

Local panels of experts from a wide variety of disciplines including general, old age, child and learning disability psychiatry and psychology. The panel will also include those with social care and mental health nursing backgrounds. Members of the panel will be of consultant grade, or, in the case of social workers or nurses, will have appropriate seniority and experience. Appointments will be made by the Commission for Mental Health.

Formal assessment

All patients coming within the provisions of the new legislation will undergo a formal assessment in accordance with the Care Programme Approach or the corresponding guidance in Wales.

"Hare" score

The score of an individual on the Psychopathy Checklist (Revised) (PCL-R). The PCL-R is a construct designed by Hare, based on Clerkey's concept of the psychopath as observed in his book "The Mask of Sanity". It is a 20 item checklist. A cut off of a score of 30 (each item can score a maximum of 2 points), the subject will be designated a psychopath for research purposes.

Hospital and limitation direction

Where the Court imposes a prison sentence at the same time as a direction of immediate admission to hospital (a hospital direction) together with a limitation direction (which has the same effect as a restriction order). When the offender is discharged from detention in hospital, he will be transferred to prison to serve the remainder of his sentence.

Information sharing

New legislation will place a duty on professionals and agencies that have responsibilities for patients who are subject to compulsory powers to share relevant information to ensure that all those involved in a patient's care and treatment are properly informed. This is often important to ensuring the patient's best interests are met, it may sometimes be necessary in the public interest.

Mental disorder

Under new legislation this will be defined to cover any disability or disorder of the mind or brain, whether permanent or temporary, which results in an impairment or disturbance of mental functioning.

Mental Health Tribunal

A new independent Tribunal will authorise the use of formal powers beyond 28 days. The Tribunal will be required to seek advice from independent experts (from the expert panel) as well as taking advice from the clinical team and hearing the views of patients or their representatives.

Mental Health National Service Framework (NSF)

Published in September 1999, the NSF has established national standards for the care and treatment of mental illness in England. An NSF for Wales is being developed in conjunction with the new All Wales Strategy for adult mental health services.

Multi Agency Risk Panels/Public Protection Panels

Local panels led by the police and probation services, and involving other agencies such as health, social services and housing, which agree local arrangements for managing the risk posed by potentially dangerous offenders in the community.

National Care Standards Commission

Provisions for the Commission were made in the Care Standards Act 2000 and it is expected to take on its regulatory responsibilities from April 2002. The Commission is an independent inspection and regulatory system for independent health and social care services.

National Oversight Group

A national group involving representatives from Regional Specialised Commissioning Groups, chaired by the NHS Executive Director of Operations, which oversees the development and operation of regional commissioning of high security psychiatric services.

Personality disorder

A disorder of the development of personality. It includes a range of mood, feeling and behavioural disorders including anti-social behaviour.

Place of safety

Any suitable place to which a person is taken under the new legislation for the purpose of carrying out a preliminary examination.

Primary Care Trusts (PCTs)

PCTs are free-standing bodies, accountable to their Health Authority for commissioning care and responsible for the provision of community services.

Psychiatric supervisor

A psychiatrist who is responsible for supervising an offender on conditional discharge from compulsory care and treatment in hospital. The psychiatric supervisor is currently known as the supervising psychiatrist.

Restriction order

When, in the case of an offender, a compulsory care and treatment order in hospital is made, the Court will be able to impose a restriction order where it appears necessary for the protection of the public from serious harm. The principal effect of the restriction order will be that the patient cannot be discharged from hospital without the consent of the Home Secretary or that of the Mental Health Tribunal in accordance with certain statutory criteria. It also means that the Home Secretary's consent is needed for the patient to be allowed out of hospital either for short periods or to move to another hospital.

Restriction direction

When transferring a prisoner from prison to hospital for compulsory care and treatment, the Home Secretary may, and in most cases will, also impose a restriction direction, so that the patient cannot be transferred to another hospital, sent on leave or discharged without his consent.

Restricted patient

A patient subject to a restriction order or restriction direction.

Second opinion approved doctor

A psychiatrist appointed by the Commission for Mental Health to provide a second opinion, as required by legislation, on the continued use of medication in the face of a patient's persistent objection or, providing the special safeguards in respect of patients with long term mental incapability who do not resist treatment. He or she also provides a second opinion on the use of treatments requiring special safeguards such as psychosurgery or the use of electro-convulsive therapy.

Social supervisor

A social worker (or in some cases, a probation officer) who is responsible for the supervision of an offender on conditional discharge from compulsory care and treatment in hospital.

Specialist mental health service

Care and treatment for a mental disorder which is provided under the management of a clinical supervisor.

Tariff

The period of a life sentence to be served to meet the requirements of retribution and deterrence before a prisoner is eligible for release on life licence.

Therapeutic benefit

The concept of therapeutic benefit will cover improvements in the symptoms of mental disorder or slowing down deterioration and the management of behaviours arising from the mental disorder.

Therapeutic community

A therapeutic community is a consciously designed social environment within a residential or day unit in which the social and group process is used for therapeutic intent. The community is the primary therapeutic instrument and provides a context for other therapies.

Transfer direction

A warrant issued by the Home Secretary, following medical recommendations, directing that a prisoner be transferred to a named psychiatric hospital for compulsory care and treatment.

'Treatability'

In the 1983 Act 'treatability' is a narrow concept that only applies to certain categories of mental disorder. In new legislation this will be framed to enable those who pose a significant risk of serious harm to others as a result of thier mental disorder to be detained in a therapeutic environment where they can be offered care and treatment.

Urgent treatment

Any treatment that needs to be provided immediately, in the best interests of the patient and which cannot await the development of a care plan.

Printed in the UK for The Stationery Office Limited
On behalf of the Controller of Her Majesty's Stationery Office
Dd 5069777 2/01 019585 589686 TJ003535 Reprinted 2001